MW00512745

The Super Tasty Mediterranean Everyday Dishes

Effortless and Inspired Recipes To Burn Fat Affordable For Beginners

Michael Anderson

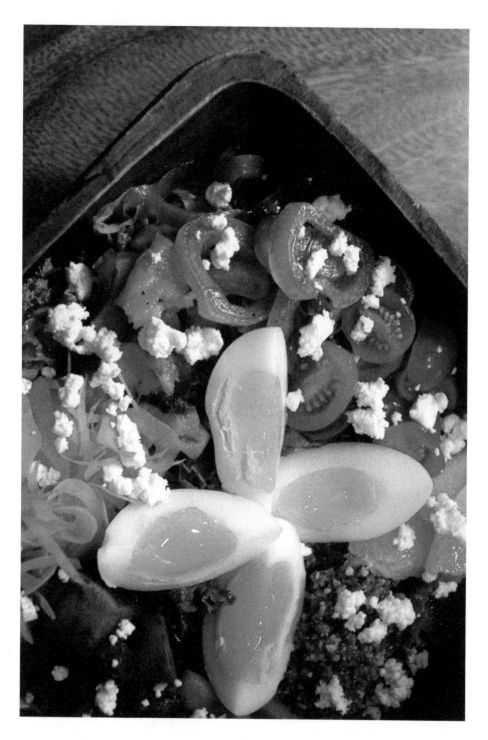

acknowledge that the author is not engaging in the rendering of legal, financial, medical or professional advice. The content within this book has been derived from various sources. Please consult a licensed professional before attempting any techniques outlined in this book.

By reading this document, the reader agrees that under no circumstances is the author responsible for any losses, direct or indirect, which are incurred as a result of the use of information contained within this document, including, but not limited to, — errors, omissions, or inaccuracies.

Table of contents

Vegetable Mains

Roasted Veggies and Brown Rice Bowl

Prep time: 15 minutes | Cook time: 20 minutes | Serves 4

2 cups cauliflower florets

2 cups broccoli florets

1 (15-ounce / 425-g) can chickpeas, drained and rinsed

1 cup carrot slices (about 1 inch thick)

2 to 3 tablespoons extra-virgin olive oil, divided

Salt and freshly ground black pepper, to taste

Nonstick cooking spray

2 cups cooked brown rice

2 to 3 tablespoons sesame seeds, for garnish

Dressing:

3 to 4 tablespoons tahini

2 tablespoons honey

1 lemon, juiced

1 garlic clove, minced

Salt and freshly ground black pepper, to taste

1. Preheat the oven to 400ºF (205ºC). Spritz two baking sheets with nonstick cooking spray.
2. Spread the cauliflower and broccoli on the first baking sheet and the second with the chickpeas and carrot slices.

3. Drizzle each sheet with half of the olive oil and sprinkle with salt and pepper. Toss to coat well.

4. Roast the chickpeas and carrot slices in the preheated oven for 10 minutes, leaving the carrots tender but crisp, and the cauliflower and broccoli for 20 minutes until fork-tender. Stir them once halfway through the cooking time.

5. Meanwhile, make the dressing: Whisk together the tahini, honey, lemon juice, garlic, salt, and pepper in a small bowl.

6. Divide the cooked brown rice among four bowls. Top each bowl evenly with roasted vegetables and dressing. Sprinkle the sesame seeds on top for garnish before serving.

Per Serving

calories: 453 | fat: 17.8g | protein: 12.1g | carbs: 61.8g | fiber: 11.2g | sodium: 60mg

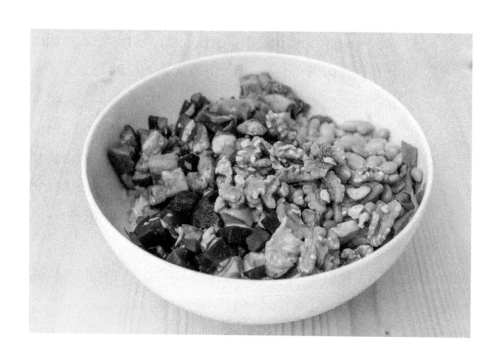

Cauliflower Hash with Carrots

Prep time: 10 minutes | Cook time: 10 minutes | Serves 4

3 tablespoons extra-virgin olive oil

1 large onion, chopped

1 tablespoon minced garlic

2 cups diced carrots

4 cups cauliflower florets

½ teaspoon ground cumin

1 teaspoon salt

1. In a large skillet, heat the olive oil over medium heat.
2. Add the onion and garlic and saut é for 1 minute. Stir in the carrots and stir-fry for 3 minutes.
3. Add the cauliflower florets, cumin, and salt and toss to combine.
4. Cover and cook for 3 minutes until lightly browned. Stir well and cook, uncovered, for 3 to 4 minutes, until softened.
5. Remove from the heat and serve warm.

Per Serving

calories: 158 | fat: 10.8g | protein: 3.1g | carbs: 14.9g | fiber: 5.1g | sodium: 656mg

Moroccan Tagine with Vegetables

Prep time: 20 minutes | Cook time: 40 minutes | Serves 2

2 tablespoons olive oil

½ onion, diced

1 garlic clove, minced

2 cups cauliflower florets

1 medium carrot, cut into 1-inch pieces

1 cup diced eggplant

1 (28-ounce / 794-g) can whole tomatoes with their juices

1 (15-ounce / 425-g) can chickpeas, drained and rinsed

2 small red potatoes, cut into 1-inch pieces

1 cup water

1 teaspoon pure maple syrup

½ teaspoon cinnamon

½ teaspoon turmeric

1 teaspoon cumin

½ teaspoon salt

1 to 2 teaspoons harissa paste

1. In a Dutch oven, heat the olive oil over medium-high heat. Sauté the onion for 5 minutes, stirring occasionally, or until the onion is translucent.

2. Stir in the garlic, cauliflower florets, carrot, eggplant, tomatoes, and potatoes. Using a

wooden spoon or spatula to break up the tomatoes into smaller pieces.

3. Add the chickpeas, water, maple syrup, cinnamon, turmeric, cumin, and salt and stir to incorporate. Bring the mixture to a boil.

4. Once it starts to boil, reduce the heat to medium-low. Stir in the harissa paste, cover, allow to simmer for about 40 minutes, or until the vegetables are softened. Taste and adjust seasoning as needed.

5. Let the mixture cool for 5 minutes before serving.

Per Serving

calories: 293 | fat: 9.9g | protein: 11.2g | carbs: 45.5g | fiber: 12.1g | sodium: 337mg

Vegan Lentil Bolognese

Prep time: 15 minutes | Cook time: 50 minutes | Serves 2

1 medium celery stalk

1 large carrot

½ large onion

1 garlic clove

2 tablespoons olive oil

1 (28-ounce / 794-g) can crushed tomatoes

1 cup red wine

½ teaspoon salt, plus more as needed

½ teaspoon pure maple syrup

1 cup cooked lentils (prepared from ½ cup dry)

1. Add the celery, carrot, onion, and garlic to a food processor and process until everything is finely chopped.
2. In a Dutch oven, heat the olive oil over medium-high heat. Add the chopped mixture and saut é for about 10 minutes, stirring occasionally, or until the vegetables are lightly browned.
3. Stir in the tomatoes, wine, salt, and maple syrup and bring to a boil.
4. Once the sauce starts to boil, cover, and reduce the heat to medium-low. Simmer for 30

minutes, stirring occasionally, or until the vegetables are softened.

5. Stir in the cooked lentils and cook for an additional 5 minutes until warmed through.

6. Taste and add additional salt, if needed. Serve warm.

Per Serving

calories: 367 | fat: 15.0g | protein: 13.7g | carbs: 44.5g | fiber: 17.6g | sodium: 1108mg

Grilled Vegetable Skewers

Prep time: 15 minutes | Cook time: 10 minutes | Serves 4

4 medium red onions, peeled and sliced into 6 wedges

4 medium zucchinis, cut into 1-inch-thick slices

2 beefsteak tomatoes, cut into quarters

4 red bell peppers, cut into 2-inch squares

2 orange bell peppers, cut into 2-inch squares

2 yellow bell peppers, cut into 2-inch squares

2 tablespoons plus

1 teaspoon olive oil, divided

Special Equipment:

4 wooden skewers, soaked in water for at least 30 minutes

1. Preheat the grill to medium-high heat.
2. Skewer the vegetables by alternating between red onion, zucchini, tomatoes, and the different colored bell peppers. Brush them with 2 tablespoons of olive oil.
3. Oil the grill grates with 1 teaspoon of olive oil and grill the vegetable skewers for 5 minutes. Flip the skewers and grill for 5 minutes more, or until they are cooked to your liking.

4. Let the skewers cool for 5 minutes before serving.

Per Serving

calories: 115 | fat: 3.0g | protein: 3.5g | carbs: 18.7g | fiber: 4.7g | sodium: 12mg

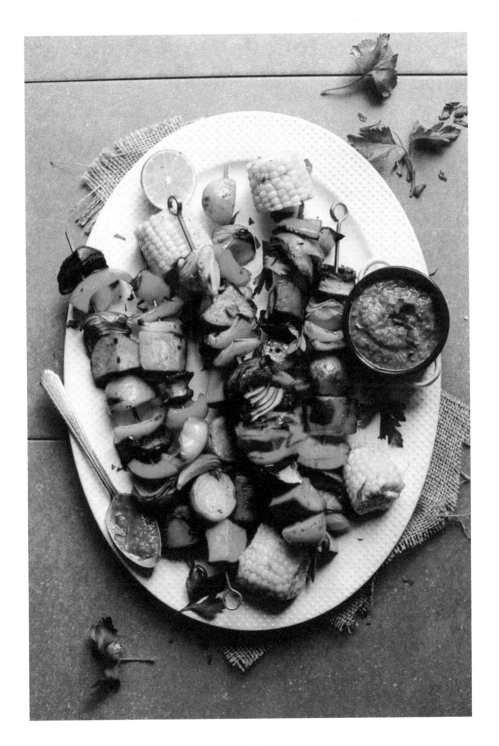

Stuffed Portobello Mushroom with Tomatoes

Prep time: 10 minutes | Cook time: 15 minutes | Serves 4

4 large portobello mushroom caps

3 tablespoons extra-virgin olive oil

Salt and freshly ground black pepper, to taste

4 sun-dried tomatoes

1 cup shredded mozzarella cheese, divided

½ to ¾ cup low-sodium tomato sauce

1. Preheat the broiler to High.
2. Arrange the mushroom caps on a baking sheet and drizzle with olive oil.
1. Sprinkle with salt and pepper.
2. Broil for 1o minutes, flipping the mushroom caps halfway through, until browned on the top.
3. Remove from the broil. Spoon 1 tomato, 2 tablespoons of cheese, and 2 to 3 tablespoons of sauce onto each mushroom cap.
4. Return the mushroom caps to the broiler and continue broiling for 2 to 3 minutes.
5. Cool for 5 minutes before serving.

Per Serving

calories: 217 | fat: 15.8g | protein: 11.2g | carbs: 11.7g | fiber: 2.0g | sodium: 243mg

Wilted Dandelion Greens with Sweet Onion

Prep time: 15 minutes | Cook time: 15 minutes | Serves 4

1 tablespoon extra-virgin olive oil

2 garlic cloves, minced

1 Vidalia onion, thinly sliced

½ cup low-sodium vegetable broth

2 bunches dandelion greens, roughly chopped

Freshly ground black pepper, to taste

1. Heat the olive oil in a large skillet over low heat.
2. Add the garlic and onion and cook for 2 to 3 minutes, stirring occasionally, or until the onion is translucent.
3. Fold in the vegetable broth and dandelion greens and cook for 5 to 7 minutes until wilted, stirring frequently.
4. Sprinkle with the black pepper and serve on a plate while warm.

Per Serving

calories: 81 | fat: 3.9g | protein: 3.2g | carbs: 10.8g | fiber: 4.0g | sodium: 72mg

Celery and Mustard Greens

Prep time: 10 minutes | Cook time: 15 minutes | Serves 4

½ cup low-sodium vegetable broth

1 celery stalk, roughly chopped

½ sweet onion, chopped

½ large red bell pepper, thinly sliced

2 garlic cloves, minced

1 bunch mustard greens, roughly chopped

1. Pour the vegetable broth into a large cast iron pan and bring it to a simmer over medium heat.
2. Stir in the celery, onion, bell pepper, and garlic. Cook uncovered for about 3 to 5 minutes, or until the onion is softened.
3. Add the mustard greens to the pan and stir well. Cover, reduce the heat to low, and cook for an additional 10 minutes, or until the liquid is evaporated and the greens are wilted.
4. Remove from the heat and serve warm.

Per Serving (1 cup)

calories: 39 | fat: 0g | protein: 3.1g | carbs: 6.8g | fiber: 3.0g | sodium: 120mg

Vegetable and Tofu Scramble

Prep time: 5 minutes | Cook time: 10 minutes | Serves 2

2 tablespoons extra-virgin olive oil

½ red onion, finely chopped

1 cup chopped kale

8 ounces (227 g) mushrooms, sliced

8 ounces (227 g) tofu, cut into pieces

2 garlic cloves, minced

Pinch red pepper flakes

½ teaspoon sea salt

⅛ teaspoon freshly ground black pepper

1. Heat the olive oil in a medium nonstick skillet over medium-high heat until shimmering.
2. Add the onion, kale, and mushrooms to the skillet and cook for about 5 minutes, stirring occasionally, or until the vegetables start to brown.
3. Add the tofu and stir-fry for 3 to 4 minutes until softened.
4. Stir in the garlic, red pepper flakes, salt, and black pepper and cook for 30 seconds.

5. Let the mixture cool for 5 minutes before serving.

Per Serving

calories: 233 | fat: 15.9g | protein: 13.4g | carbs: 11.9g | fiber: 2.0g | sodium: 672mg

Zoodles

Prep time: 10 minutes | Cook time: 5 minutes | Serves 2

2 tablespoons avocado oil

2 medium zucchini, spiralized

¼ teaspoon salt

Freshly ground black pepper, to taste

1. Heat the avocado oil in a large skillet over medium heat until it shimmers.
2. Add the zucchini noodles, salt, and black pepper to the skillet and toss to coat. Cook for 1 to 2 minutes, stirring constantly, until tender.
3. Serve warm.

Per Serving

calories: 128 | fat: 14.0g | protein: 0.3g | carbs: 0.3g | fiber: 0.1g | sodium: 291mg

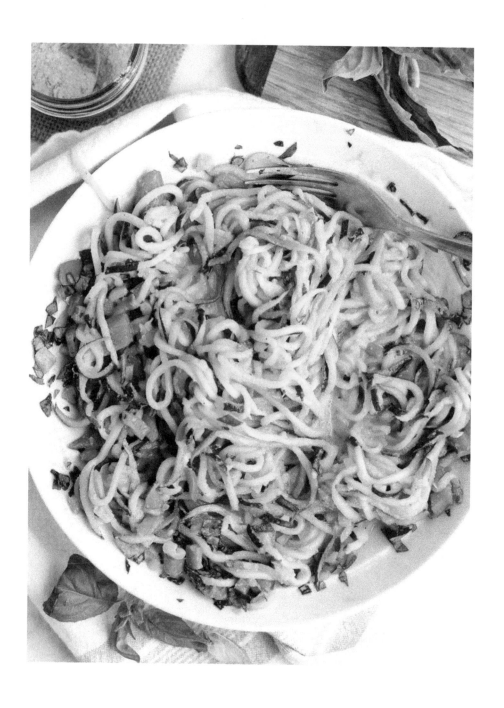

Lentil and Tomato Collard Wraps

Prep time: 15 minutes | Cook time: 0 minutes | Serves 4

2 cups cooked lentils

5 Roma tomatoes, diced

½ cup crumbled feta cheese

10 large fresh basil leaves, thinly sliced

¼ cup extra-virgin olive oil

1 tablespoon balsamic vinegar

2 garlic cloves, minced

½ teaspoon raw honey

½ teaspoon salt

¼ teaspoon freshly ground black pepper

4 large collard leaves, stems removed

1. Combine the lentils, tomatoes, cheese, basil leaves, olive oil, vinegar, garlic, honey, salt, and black pepper in a large bowl and stir until well blended.
2. Lay the collard leaves on a flat work surface. Spoon the equal-sized amounts of the lentil mixture onto the edges of the leaves. Roll them up and slice in half to serve.

Per Serving

calories: 318 | fat: 17.6g | protein: 13.2g | carbs: 27.5g | fiber: 9.9g | sodium: 475mg

Stir-Fry Baby Bok Choy

Prep time: 12 minutes | Cook time: 10 to 13 minutes | Serves 6

2 tablespoons coconut oil

1 large onion, finely diced

2 teaspoons ground cumin

1-inch piece fresh ginger, grated

1 teaspoon ground turmeric

½ teaspoon salt

12 baby bok choy heads, ends trimmed and sliced lengthwise

Water, as needed

3 cups cooked brown rice

1. Heat the coconut oil in a large pan over medium heat.
2. Sauté the onion for 5 minutes, stirring occasionally, or until the onion is translucent.
3. Fold in the cumin, ginger, turmeric, and salt and stir to coat well.
4. Add the bok choy and cook for 5 to 8 minutes, stirring occasionally, or until the bok choy is tender but crisp. You can add 1 tablespoon of

water at a time, if the skillet gets dry until you finish sautéing.

5. Transfer the bok choy to a plate and serve over the cooked brown rice.

Per Serving

calories: 443 | fat: 8.8g | protein: 30.3g | carbs: 75.7g | fiber: 19.0g | sodium: 1289mg

Sweet Pepper Stew

Prep time: 20 minutes | Cook time: 50 minutes | Serves 2

2 tablespoons olive oil

2 sweet peppers, diced (about 2 cups)

½ large onion, minced

1 garlic clove, minced

1 tablespoon gluten-free Worcestershire sauce

1 teaspoon oregano

1 cup low-sodium tomato juice

1 cup low-sodium vegetable stock

¼ cup brown rice

¼ cup brown lentils

Salt, to taste

1. In a Dutch oven, heat the olive oil over medium-high heat.
2. Saut é the sweet peppers and onion for 10 minutes, stirring occasionally, or until the onion begins to turn golden and the peppers are wilted.
3. Stir in the garlic, Worcestershire sauce, and oregano and cook for 30 seconds more. Add the tomato juice, vegetable stock, rice, and lentils to the Dutch oven and stir to mix well.
4. Bring the mixture to a boil and then reduce the heat to medium-low. Let it simmer covered for

about 45 minutes, or until the rice is cooked through and the lentils are tender.

5. Sprinkle with salt and serve warm.

Per Serving

calories: 378 | fat: 15.6g | protein: 11.4g | carbs: 52.8g | fiber: 7.0g | sodium: 391mg

Fish and Seafood

Salmon Baked in Foil

Prep time: 5 minutes | Cook time: 25 minutes | Serves 4

2 cups cherry tomatoes

3 tablespoons extra-virgin olive oil

3 tablespoons lemon juice

3 tablespoons almond butter

1 teaspoon oregano

½ teaspoon salt

4 (5-ounce / 142-g) salmon fillets

1. Preheat the oven to 400ºF (205ºC).
2. Cut the tomatoes in half and put them in a bowl.
3. Add the olive oil, lemon juice, butter, oregano, and salt to the tomatoes and gently toss to combine.
4. Cut 4 pieces of foil, about 12-by-12 inches each.
5. Place the salmon fillets in the middle of each piece of foil.
6. Divide the tomato mixture evenly over the 4 pieces of salmon. Bring the ends of the foil together and seal to form a closed pocket.

7. Place the 4 pockets on a baking sheet. Bake in the preheated oven for 25 minutes.

8. Remove from the oven and serve on a plate.

Per Serving

calories: 410 | fat: 32.0g | protein: 30.0g | carbs: 4.0g | fiber: 1.0g | sodium: 370mg

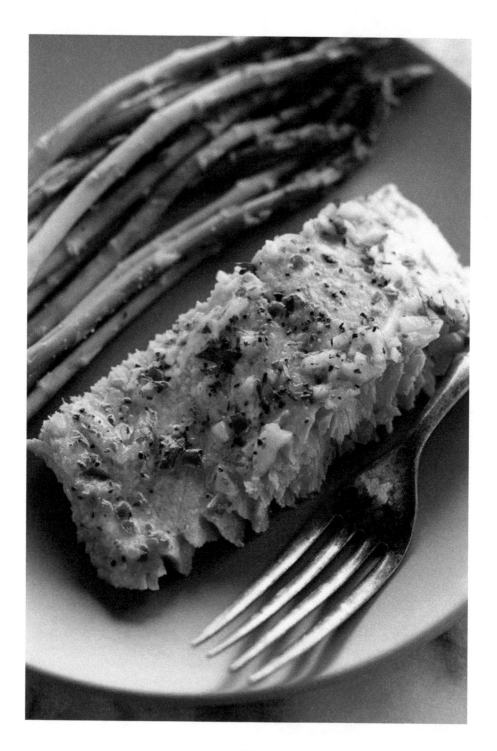

Instant Pot Poached Salmon

Prep time: 10 minutes | Cook time: 3 minutes | Serves 4

1 lemon, sliced ¼ inch thick

4 (6-ounce / 170-g) skinless salmon fillets, 1½ inches thick

½ teaspoon salt

¼ teaspoon pepper

½ cup water

1. Layer the lemon slices in the bottom of the Instant Pot.
2. Season the salmon with salt and pepper, then arrange the salmon (skin- side down) on top of the lemon slices. Pour in the water.
3. Secure the lid. Select the Manual mode and set the cooking time for 3 minutes at High Pressure.
4. Once cooking is complete, do a quick pressure release. Carefully open the lid.
5. Serve warm.

Per Serving

calories: 350 | fat: 23.0g | protein: 35.0g | carbs: 0g | fiber: 0g | sodium: 390mg

Balsamic-Honey Glazed Salmon

Prep time: 2 minutes | Cook time: 8 minutes | Serves 4

½ cup balsamic vinegar

1 tablespoon honey

4 (8-ounce / 227-g) salmon fillets

Sea salt and freshly ground pepper, to taste

1 tablespoon olive oil

1. Heat a skillet over medium-high heat. Combine the vinegar and honey in a small bowl.
2. Season the salmon fillets with the sea salt and freshly ground pepper; brush with the honey-balsamic glaze.
3. Add olive oil to the skillet, and sear the salmon fillets, cooking for 3 to 4 minutes on each side until lightly browned and medium rare in the center.
4. Let sit for 5 minutes before serving.

Per Serving

calories: 454 | fat: 17.3g | protein: 65.3g | carbs: 9.7g | fiber: 0g | sodium: 246mg

Seared Salmon with Lemon Cream Sauce

Prep time: 10 minutes | Cook time: 20 minutes | Serves 4

4 (5-ounce / 142-g) salmon fillets

Sea salt and freshly ground black pepper, to taste

1 tablespoon extra-virgin olive oil

½ cup low-sodium vegetable broth

Juice and zest of 1 lemon

1 teaspoon chopped fresh thyme

½ cup fat-free sour cream

1 teaspoon honey

1 tablespoon chopped fresh chives

1. Preheat the oven to 400ºF (205ºC).
2. Season the salmon lightly on both sides with salt and pepper.
3. Place a large ovenproof skillet over medium-high heat and add the olive oil.
4. Sear the salmon fillets on both sides until golden, about 3 minutes per side.
5. Transfer the salmon to a baking dish and bake in the preheated oven until just cooked through, about 10 minutes.

6. Meanwhile, whisk together the vegetable broth, lemon juice and zest, and thyme in a small saucepan over medium-high heat until the liquid reduces by about one-quarter, about 5 minutes.
7. Whisk in the sour cream and honey.
8. Stir in the chives and serve the sauce over the salmon.

Per Serving

calories: 310 | fat: 18.0g | protein: 29.0g | carbs: 6.0g | fiber: 0g | sodium: 129mg

Tuna and Zucchini Patties

Prep time: 10 minutes | Cook time: 12 minutes | Serves 4

3 slices whole-wheat sandwich bread, toasted

2 (5-ounce / 142-g) cans tuna in olive oil, drained

1 cup shredded zucchini

1 large egg, lightly beaten

¼ cup diced red bell pepper

1 tablespoon dried oregano

1 teaspoon lemon zest

¼ teaspoon freshly ground black pepper

¼ teaspoon kosher or sea salt

1 tablespoon extra-virgin olive oil

Salad greens or 4 whole-wheat rolls, for serving (optional)

1. Crumble the toast into bread crumbs with your fingers (or use a knife to cut into ¼-inch cubes) until you have 1 cup of loosely packed crumbs. Pour the crumbs into a large bowl. Add the tuna, zucchini, beaten egg, bell pepper, oregano, lemon zest, black pepper, and salt. Mix well with a fork. With your hands, form the mixture into four (½-cup-size) patties. Place

them on a plate, and press each patty flat to about ¾-inch thick.

2. In a large skillet over medium-high heat, heat the oil until it's very hot, about 2 minutes.

3. Add the patties to the hot oil, then reduce the heat down to medium. Cook the patties for 5 minutes, flip with a spatula, and cook for an additional 5 minutes. Serve the patties on salad greens or whole-wheat rolls, if desired.

Per Serving

calories: 757 | fat: 72.0g | protein: 5.0g | carbs: 26.0g | fiber: 4.0g | sodium: 418mg

Fennel Poached Cod with Tomatoes

Prep time: 10 minutes | Cook time: 20 minutes | Serves 4

1 tablespoon olive oil

1 cup thinly sliced fennel

½ cup thinly sliced onion

1 tablespoon minced garlic

1 (15-ounce / 425-g) can diced tomatoes

2 cups chicken broth

½ cup white wine

Juice and zest of 1 orange

1 pinch red pepper flakes

1 bay leaf

1 pound (454 g) cod

1. Heat the olive oil in a large skillet. Add the onion and fennel and cook for 6 minutes, stirring occasionally, or until translucent. Add the garlic and cook for 1 minute more.
2. Add the tomatoes, chicken broth, wine, orange juice and zest, red pepper flakes, and bay leaf, and simmer for 5 minutes to meld the flavors.
3. Carefully add the cod in a single layer, cover, and simmer for 6 to 7 minutes.

4. Transfer fish to a serving dish, ladle the remaining sauce over the fish, and serve.

Per Serving

calories: 336 | fat: 12.5g | protein: 45.1g | carbs:11.0g | fiber: 3.3g | sodium: 982mg

Teriyaki Salmon

Prep time: 10 minutes | Cook time: 8 minutes | Serves 4

4 (8-ounce / 227-g) thick salmon fillets.

1 cup soy sauce

2 cups water

½ cup mirin

2 tablespoons sesame oil

4 teaspoons sesame seeds

2 cloves garlic, minced

2 tablespoons freshly grated ginger

4 tablespoons brown sugar

1 tablespoon corn starch

4 green onions, minced

1. Add the soy sauce, sesame oil, sesame seeds, mirin, ginger, water, garlic, green onions, and brown sugar to a small bowl. Mix them well.
2. In a shallow dish place the salmon fillets and pour half of the prepared mixture over the fillets. Let it marinate for 30 minutes in a refrigerator.
3. Pour 1 cup of water into the insert of your Instant pot and place trivet inside it.

4. Arrange the marinated salmon fillets over the trivet and secure the lid.

5. Select the Manual settings with High Pressure and 8 minutes cooking time.

6. Meanwhile, take a skillet and add the remaining marinade mixture in it.

7. Let it cook for 2 minutes, then add the corn starch mixed with water. Stir well and cook for 1 minute.

8. Check the pressure cooker, do a Quick release if it is done.

9. Transfer the fillets to a serving platter and pour the sesame mixture over it.

10. Garnish with chopped green chilies then serve hot.

Per Serving

calories: 622 | fat: 28.6g | protein: 51.3g | carbs: 29.6g | fiber: 2.0g | sodium: 1086mg

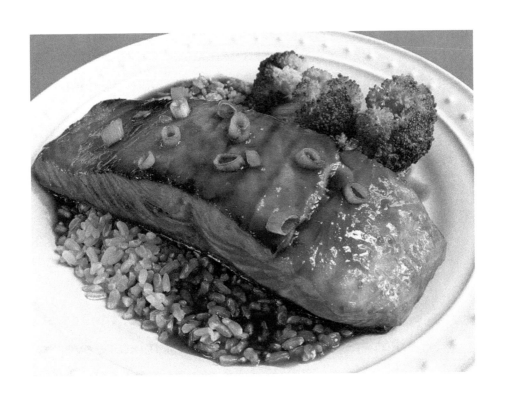

Coconut Tangy Cod Curry

Prep time: 5 minutes | Cook time: 3 minutes | Serves 6

1 (28-ounce / 794-g) can coconut milk

Juice of 2 lemons

2 tablespoons red curry paste

2 teaspoons fish sauce

2 teaspoons honey

4 teaspoons Sriracha

4 cloves garlic, minced

2 teaspoons ground turmeric

2 teaspoons ground ginger

1 teaspoon sea salt

1 teaspoon white pepper

2 pounds (907 g) codfish, cut into 1-inch cubes

½ cup chopped fresh cilantro, for garnish

4 lime wedges, for garnish

1. Add all the ingredients, except the cod cubes and garnish, to a large bowl and whisk them well.

2. Arrange the cod cube at the base of the Instant Pot and pour the coconut milk mixture over it.

3. Secure the lid and hit the Manual key, select High Pressure with 3 minutes cooking time.

4. After the beep, do a Quick release then remove the lid.

5. Garnish with fresh cilantro and lemon wedges then serve.

Per Serving

calories: 396 | fat: 29.1g | protein: 26.6g | carbs: 11.4g | fiber: 2.0g | sodium: 1024mg

Shrimps with Broccoli

Prep time: 5 minutes | Cook time: 10 minutes | Serves 2

2 teaspoons vegetable oil

2 tablespoons corn starch

1 cup broccoli florets

¼ cup chicken broth

8 ounces (227 g) large shrimp, peeled and deveined

¼ cup soy sauce

¼ cup water

¼ cup sliced carrots

3 tablespoons rice vinegar

2 teaspoons sesame oil

1 tablespoon chili garlic sauce

Coriander leaves to garnish

Boiled rice or noodles, for serving

1. Add 1 tablespoon of corn starch and shrimp to a bowl. Mix them well then set it aside.
2. In a small bowl, mix the remaining corn starch, chicken broth, carrots, chili garlic sauce, rice vinegar and soy sauce together. Keep the mixture aside.

3. Select the Sauté function on your Instant pot, add the sesame oil and broccoli florets to the pot and sauté for 5 minutes.
4. Add the water to the broccoli, cover the lid and cook for 5 minutes.
5. Stir in shrimp and vegetable oil to the broccoli, sauté it for 5 minutes.
6. Garnish with coriander leaves on top.
7. Serve with rice or noodles.

Per Serving

calories: 300 | fat: 16.5g | protein: 19.6g | carbs: 17.1g | fiber: 2.2g | sodium: 1241mg

Sauces, Dips, and Dressings

Hot Pepper Sauce

Prep time: 10 minutes | Cook time: 20 minutes | Makes 4 cups

1 red hot fresh chiles, deseeded

½ small yellow onion, roughly chopped

2 dried chiles

2 cups water

2 garlic cloves, peeled

2 cups white vinegar

1. Place all the ingredients except the vinegar in a medium saucepan over medium heat. Allow to simmer for 20 minutes until softened.
2. Transfer the mixture to a food processor or blender. Stir in the vinegar and pulse until very smooth.
3. Serve immediately or transfer to a sealed container and refrigerate for up to 3 months.

Per Serving (2 tablespoons)

calories: 20 | fat: 1.2g | protein: 0.6g | carbs: 4.4g | fiber: 0.6g | sodium: 12mg

Lemon-Tahini Sauce

Prep time: 10 minutes | Cook time: 0 minutes | Makes 1 cup

½ cup tahini

1 garlic clove, minced

Juice and zest of 1 lemon

½ teaspoon salt, plus more as needed

½ cup warm water, plus more as needed

1. Combine the tahini and garlic in a small bowl.
2. Add the lemon juice and zest and salt to the bowl and stir to mix well.
3. Fold in the warm water and whisk until well combined and creamy. Feel free to add more warm water if you like a thinner consistency.
4. Taste and add more salt as needed.
5. Store the sauce in a sealed container in the refrigerator for up to 5 days.

Per Serving (¼ cup)

calories: 179 | fat: 15.5g | protein: 5.1g | carbs: 6.8g | fiber: 3.0g | sodium: 324mg

Peri-Peri Sauce

Prep time: 10 minutes | Cook time: 5 minutes | Serves 4

1 tomato, chopped

1 red onion, chopped

1 red bell pepper, deseeded and chopped

1 red chile, deseeded and chopped

4 garlic cloves, minced

2 tablespoons extra-virgin olive oil

Juice of 1 lemon

1 tablespoon dried oregano

1 tablespoon smoked paprika

1 teaspoon sea salt

1. Process all the ingredients in a food processor or a blender until smooth.
2. Transfer the mixture to a small saucepan over medium-high heat and bring to a boil, stirring often.
3. Reduce the heat to medium and allow to simmer for 5 minutes until heated through.
4. You can store the sauce in an airtight container in the refrigerator for up to 5 days.

Per Serving

calories: 98 | fat: 6.5g | protein: 1.0g | carbs: 7.8g | fiber: 3.0g | sodium: 295mg

Peanut Sauce with Honey

Prep time: 5 minutes | Cook time: 0 minutes | Serves 4

¼ cup peanut butter

1 tablespoon peeled and grated fresh ginger

1 tablespoon honey

1 tablespoon low-sodium soy sauce

1 garlic clove, minced

Juice of 1 lime

Pinch red pepper flakes

1. Whisk together all the ingredients in a small bowl until well incorporated.
2. Transfer to an airtight container and refrigerate for up to 5 days.

Per Serving

calories: 117 | fat: 7.6g | protein: 4.1g | carbs: 8.8g | fiber: 1.0g | sodium: 136mg

Cilantro-Tomato Salsa

Prep time: 10 minutes | Cook time: 0 minutes | Serves 6

2 or 3 medium, ripe tomatoes, diced

1 serrano pepper, seeded and minced

½ red onion, minced

¼ cup minced fresh cilantro

Juice of 1 lime

¼ teaspoon salt, plus more as needed

1. Place the tomatoes, serrano pepper, onion, cilantro, lime juice, and salt in a small bowl and mix well.
2. Taste and add additional salt, if needed.
3. Store in an airtight container in the refrigerator for up to 3 days.

Per Serving (¼ cup)

calories: 17 | fat: 0g | protein: 1.0g | carbs: 3.9g | fiber: 1.0g | sodium: 83mg

Cheesy Pea Pesto

Prep time: 5 minutes | Cook time: 0 minutes | Serves 4

½ cup fresh green peas

¼ cup pine nuts

½ cup grated Parmesan cheese

¼ cup fresh basil leaves

¼ cup extra-virgin olive oil

2 garlic cloves, minced

¼ teaspoon sea salt

1. Add all the ingredients to a food processor or blender and pulse until the nuts are chopped finely.
2. Transfer to an airtight container and refrigerate for up to 2 days. You can also store it in ice cube trays in the freezer for up to 6 months.

Per Serving

calories: 247 | fat: 22.8g | protein: 7.1g | carbs: 4.8g | fiber: 1.0g | sodium: 337mg

Guacamole

Prep time: 10 minutes | Cook time: 0 minutes | Serves 6

2 large avocados

¼ white onion, finely diced

1 small, firm tomato, finely diced

¼ cup finely chopped fresh cilantro

2 tablespoons freshly squeezed lime juice

¼ teaspoon salt

Freshly ground black pepper, to taste

1. Slice the avocados in half and remove the pits. Using a large spoon to scoop out the flesh and add to a medium bowl.
2. Mash the avocado flesh with the back of a fork, or until a uniform consistency is achieved. Add the onion, tomato, cilantro, lime juice, salt, and pepper to the bowl and stir to combine.
3. Serve immediately, or transfer to an airtight container and refrigerate until chilled.

Per Serving (¼ cup)

calories: 81 | fat: 6.8g | protein: 1.1g | carbs: 5.7g | fiber: 3.0g | sodium: 83mg

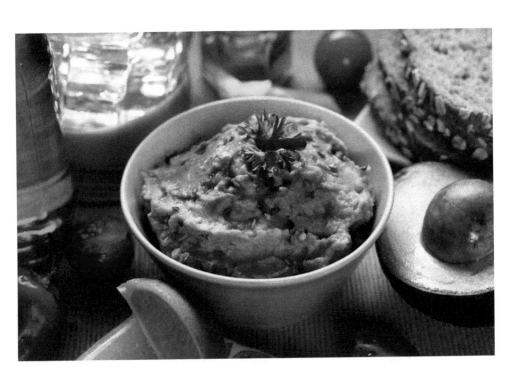

Lentil-Tahini Dip

Prep time: 10 minutes | Cook time: 15 minutes | Makes 3 cups

1 cup dried green or brown lentils, rinsed

2½ cups water, divided

1⅃ cup tahini

1 garlic clove

½ teaspoon salt, plus more as needed

1. Add the lentils and 2 cups of water to a medium saucepan and bring to a boil over high heat.
2. Once it starts to boil, reduce the heat to low, and then cook for 14 minutes, stirring occasionally, or the lentils become tender but still hold their shape. You can drain any excess liquid.
3. Transfer the lentils to a food processor, along with the remaining water, tahini, garlic, and salt and process until smooth and creamy.
4. Taste and adjust the seasoning if needed. Serve immediately.

Per Serving (¼ cup)

calories: 100 | fat: 3.9g | protein: 5.1g | carbs: 10.7g | fiber: 6.0g | sodium: 106mg

Lemon-Dill Cashew Dip

Prep time: 10 minutes | Cook time: 0 minutes | Makes 1 cup

¾ cup cashews, soaked in water for at least 4 hours and drained well

¼ cup water

Juice and zest of 1 lemon

2 tablespoons chopped fresh dill

¼ teaspoon salt, plus more as needed

1. Put the cashews, water, lemon juice and zest in a blender and blend until smooth.
2. Add the dill and salt to the blender and blend again.
3. Taste and adjust the seasoning, if needed.
4. Transfer to an airtight container and refrigerate for at least 1 hour to blend the flavors.
5. Serve chilled.

Per Serving (1 tablespoon)

calories: 37 | fat: 2.9g | protein: 1.1g | carbs: 1.9g | fiber: 0g | sodium: 36mg

Homemade Blackened Seasoning

Prep time: 10 minutes | Cook time: 0 minutes | Makes about ½ cup

2 tablespoons smoked paprika

2 tablespoons garlic powder

2 tablespoons onion powder

1 tablespoon sweet paprika

1 teaspoon dried dill

1 teaspoon freshly ground black pepper

½ teaspoon ground mustard

¼ teaspoon celery seeds

1. Add all the ingredients to a small bowl and mix well.
2. Serve immediately, or transfer to an airtight container and store in a cool, dry and dark place for up to 3 months.

Per Serving (1 tablespoon)

calories: 22 | fat: 0.9g | protein: 1.0g | carbs: 4.7g | fiber: 1.0g | sodium: 2mg

Breakfast

Greek Yogurt with Fresh Berries, Honey and Nuts

Preparation Time: 5 minutes

Cooking Time: 0 minutes

Servings: 1

Ingredients:

- 6 oz. nonfat plain Greek yogurt
- 1/2 cup fresh berries of your choice
- 1 tbsp .25 oz crushed walnuts
- 1 tbsp honey

Directions:

1. In a jar with a lid, add the yogurt. Top with berries and a drizzle of honey. Top with the lid and store in the fridge for 2-3 days.

Nutrition:

Calories:250

Carbs: 35

Fat: 4g

Protein: 19g

Mediterranean Egg Muffins with Ham

Preparation Time: 15 minutes

Cooking Time: 15 minutes

Servings: 6

Ingredients:

- 9 Slices of thin cut deli ham
- 1/2 cup canned roasted red pepper, sliced + additional for garnish
- 1/3 cup fresh spinach, minced
- 1/4 cup feta cheese, crumbled
- 5 large eggs
- Pinch of salt
- Pinch of pepper
- 1 1/2 tbsp Pesto sauce
- Fresh basil for garnish

Directions:

1. Preheat oven to 400 degrees F. Spray a muffin tin with cooking spray, generously. Line each of the muffin tin with 1 ½ pieces of ham - making sure there aren't any holes for the egg mixture come out.

2. Place some of the roasted red pepper in the bottom of each muffin tin. Place 1 tbsp of minced spinach on top of each red pepper. Top the pepper and

71

spinach off with a large 1/2 tbsp of crumbled feta cheese.

3. In a medium bowl, whisk together the eggs salt and pepper, divide the egg mixture evenly among the 6 muffin tins.

4. Bake for 15 to 17 minutes until the eggs are puffy and set. Remove each cup from the muffin tin. Allow to cool completely

5. Distribute the muffins among the containers, store in the fridge for 2 - 3days or in the freezer for 3 months.

Nutrition:

Calories:109; Carbs: 2g; Fat: 6g; Protein: 9g

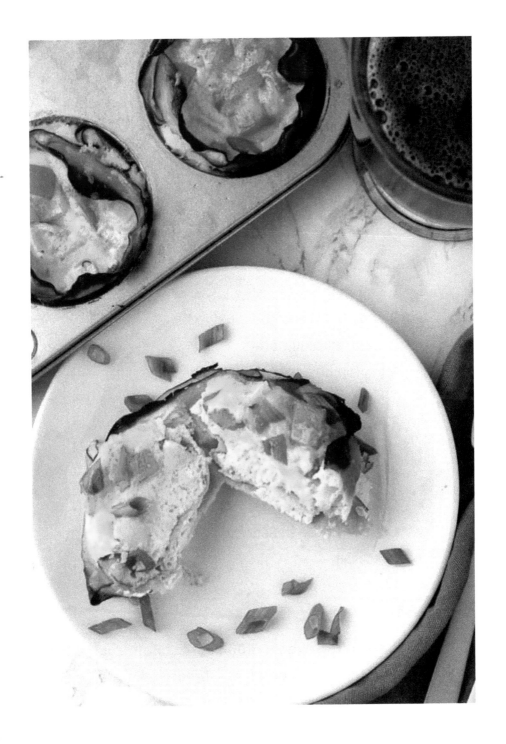

Italian Breakfast Sausage with Baby Potatoes and Vegetables

Preparation Time: 15 minutes

Cooking Time: 30 minutes

Servings: 4

Ingredients:

- 1 lb. sweet Italian sausage links, sliced on the bias (diagonal)
- 2 cups baby potatoes, halved
- 2 cups broccoli florets
- 1 cup onions cut to 1-inch chunks
- 2 cups small mushrooms -half or quarter the large ones for uniform size
- 1 cup baby carrots
- 2 tbsp olive oil
- 1/2 tsp garlic powder
- 1/2 tsp Italian seasoning
- 1 tsp salt
- 1/2 tsp pepper

Directions:

1. Preheat the oven to 400 degrees F. In a large bowl, add the baby potatoes, broccoli florets, onions, small mushrooms, and baby carrots.

2. Add in the olive oil, salt, pepper, garlic powder and Italian seasoning and toss to evenly coat. Spread the vegetables onto a sheet pan in one even layer.

3. Arrange the sausage slices on the pan over the vegetables. Bake for 30 minutes – make sure to sake halfway through to prevent sticking. Allow to cool.

4. Distribute the Italian sausages and vegetables among the containers and store in the fridge for 2-3 days

Nutrition:

Calories:321, Fat: 16g, Carbs: 23g, Protein: 22g

Sun dried Tomatoes, Dill and Feta Omelet Casserole

Preparation Time: 15 minutes

Cooking Time: 40 minutes

Servings: 6

Ingredients:

- 12 large eggs
- 2 cups whole milk
- 8 oz fresh spinach
- 2 cloves garlic, minced
- 12 oz artichoke salad with olives and peppers, drained and chopped
- 5 oz sun dried tomato feta cheese, crumbled
- 1 tbsp fresh chopped dill or 1 tsp dried dill
- 1 tsp dried oregano
- 1 tsp lemon pepper
- 1 tsp salt
- 4 tsp olive oil, divided

Directions:

1. Preheat oven to 375 degrees F. Chop the fresh herbs and artichoke salad. In a skillet over medium heat, add 1 tbsp olive oil.

2. Sauté the spinach and garlic until wilted, about 3 minutes. Oil a 9x13 inch baking dish, layer the spinach and artichoke salad evenly in the dish

3. In a medium bowl, whisk together the eggs, milk, herbs, salt and lemon pepper. Pour the egg mixture over vegetables, sprinkle with feta cheese.

4. Bake in the center of the oven for 35-40 minutes until firm in the center. Allow to cool, slice a and distribute among the storage containers. Store for 2-3 days or freeze for 3 months

Nutrition:

Calories:196, Carbohydrates: 5g, Fat: 12g, Protein: 10g

Mediterranean Breakfast Egg White Sandwich

Preparation Time: 15 minutes

Cooking Time: 30 minutes

Servings: 1

Ingredients:

- 1 tsp vegan butter
- ¼ cup egg whites
- 1 tsp chopped fresh herbs such as parsley, basil, rosemary
- 1 whole grain seeded ciabatta roll
- 1 tbsp pesto
- 1-2 slices muenster cheese (or other cheese such as provolone, Monterey Jack, etc.)
- About ½ cup roasted tomatoes
- Salt, to taste
- Pepper, to taste
- Roasted Tomatoes:
- 10 oz grape tomatoes
- 1 tbsp extra virgin olive oil
- Kosher salt, to taste
- Coarse black pepper, to taste

Directions:

1. In a small nonstick skillet over medium heat, melt the vegan butter. Pour in egg whites, season with salt and pepper, sprinkle with fresh herbs, cook for 3-4 minutes or until egg is done, flip once.
2. In the meantime, toast the ciabatta bread in toaster. Once done, spread both halves with pesto.
3. Place the egg on the bottom half of sandwich roll, folding if necessary, top with cheese, add the roasted tomatoes and top half of roll sandwich.
4. For the roasted tomatoes, preheat oven to 400 degrees F. Slice tomatoes in half lengthwise. Then place them onto a baking sheet and drizzle with the olive oil, toss to coat.
5. Season with salt and pepper and roast in oven for about 20 minutes, until the skin appears wrinkled

Nutrition:

Calories:458; Carbohydrates: 51g; Fat: 0g; Protein: 21g

Breakfast Taco Scramble

Preparation Time: 15 minutes

Cooking Time: 1 hour & 25 minutes

Servings: 4

Ingredients:

- 8 large eggs, beaten
- 1/4 tsp seasoning salt
- 1 lb. 99% lean ground turkey
- 2 tbsp Greek seasoning
- 1/2 small onion, minced
- 2 tbsp bell pepper, minced
- 4 oz. can tomato sauce
- 1/4 cup water
- 1/4 cup chopped scallions or cilantro, for topping
- For the potatoes:
- 12 (1 lb.) baby gold or red potatoes, quartered
- 4 tsp olive oil
- 3/4 tsp salt
- 1/2 tsp garlic powder
- fresh black pepper, to taste

Directions:

1. In a large bowl, beat the eggs, season with seasoning salt. Preheat the oven to 425 degrees F.

Spray a 9x12 or large oval casserole dish with cooking oil.

2. Add the potatoes 1 tbsp oil, 3/4 teaspoon salt, garlic powder and black pepper and toss to coat. Bake for 45 minutes to 1 hour, tossing every 15 minutes.

3. In the meantime, brown the turkey in a large skillet over medium heat, breaking it up while it cooks. Once no longer pink, add in the Greek seasoning.

4. Add in the bell pepper, onion, tomato sauce and water, stir and cover, simmer on low for about 20 minutes. Spray a different skillet with nonstick spray over medium heat.

5. Once heated, add in the eggs seasoned with 1/4 tsp of salt and scramble for 2–3 minutes, or cook until it sets.

6. Distribute 3/4 cup turkey and 2/3 cup eggs and divide the potatoes in each storage container, store for 3-4 days.

Nutrition:

Calories:450; Fat: 19g; Carbs: 24.5g; Protein: 46g

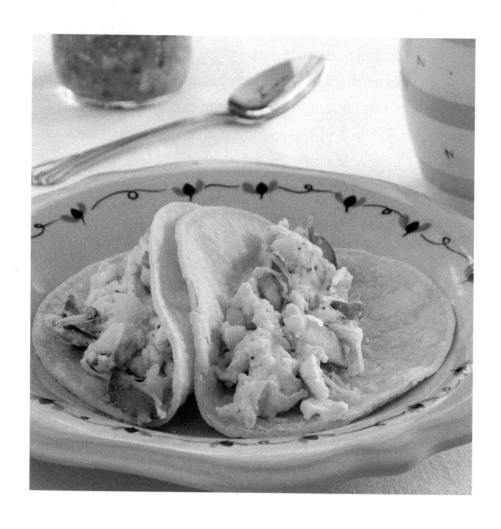

Blueberry Greek Yogurt Pancakes

Preparation Time: 15 minutes

Cooking Time: 15 minutes

Servings: 6

Ingredients:

- 1 1/4 cup all-purpose flour
- 2 tsp baking powder
- 1 tsp baking soda
- 1/4 tsp salt
- 1/4 cup sugar
- 3 eggs
- 3 tbsp vegan butter unsalted, melted
- 1/2 cup milk
- 1 1/2 cups Greek yogurt plain, non-fat
- 1/2 cup blueberries optional
- Toppings:
- Greek yogurt
- Mixed berries – blueberries, raspberries and blackberries

Directions:

1. In a large bowl, whisk together the flour, salt, baking powder and baking soda. In a separate bowl, whisk together butter, sugar, eggs, Greek yogurt, and milk until the mixture is smooth.

2. Then add in the Greek yogurt mixture from step to the dry mixture in step 1, mix to combine, allow the patter to sit for 20 minutes to get a smooth texture – if using blueberries fold them into the pancake batter.

3. Heat the pancake griddle, spray with non-stick butter spray or just brush with butter. Pour the batter, in 1/4 cupful's, onto the griddle.

4. Cook until the bubbles on top burst and create small holes, lift up the corners of the pancake to see if they're golden browned on the bottom

5. With a wide spatula, flip the pancake and cook on the other side until lightly browned. Serve.

Nutrition:

Calories:258, Carbohydrates: 33g, Fat: 8g, Protein: 11g

Cauliflower Fritters with Hummus

Preparation Time: 15 minutes

Cooking Time: 15 minutes

Servings: 4

Ingredients:

- 2 (15 oz) cans chickpeas, divided
- 2 1/2 tbsp olive oil, divided, plus more for frying
- 1 cup onion, chopped, about 1/2 a small onion
- 2 tbsp garlic, minced
- 2 cups cauliflower, cut into small pieces, about 1/2 a large head
- 1/2 tsp salt
- black pepper
- Topping:
- Hummus, of choice
- Green onion, diced

Directions:

1. Preheat oven to 400°F. Rinse and drain 1 can of the chickpeas, place them on a paper towel to dry off well.

2. Then place the chickpeas into a large bowl, removing the loose skins that come off, and toss

with 1 tbsp of olive oil, spread the chickpeas onto a large pan and sprinkle with salt and pepper.

3. Bake for 20 minutes, then stir, and then bake an additional 5-10 minutes until very crispy.

4. Once the chickpeas are roasted, transfer them to a large food processor and process until broken down and crumble - Don't over process them and turn it into flour, as you need to have some texture. Place the mixture into a small bowl, set aside.

5. In a large pan over medium-high heat, add the remaining 1 1/2 tbsp of olive oil. Once heated, add in the onion and garlic, cook until lightly golden brown, about 2 minutes.

6. Then add in the chopped cauliflower, cook for an additional 2 minutes, until the cauliflower is golden.

7. Turn the heat down to low and cover the pan, cook until the cauliflower is fork tender and the onions are golden brown and caramelized, stirring often, about 3-5 minutes.

8. Transfer the cauliflower mixture to the food processor, drain and rinse the remaining can of chickpeas and add them into the food processor, along with the salt and a pinch of pepper.

9. Blend until smooth, and the mixture starts to ball, stop to scrape down the sides as needed

10. Transfer the cauliflower mixture into a large bowl and add in 1/2 cup of the roasted chickpea crumbs, stir until well combined.

11. In a large bowl over medium heat, add in enough oil to lightly cover the bottom of a large pan. Working in batches, cook the patties until golden brown, about 2-3 minutes, flip and cook again. Serve.

Nutrition:

Calories:333

Carbohydrates: 45g

Fat: 13g

Protein: 14g

Overnight Berry Chia Oats

Preparation Time: 15 minutes

Cooking Time: 5 minutes

Servings: 1

Ingredients:

- 1/2 cup Quaker Oats rolled oats
- 1/4 cup chia seeds
- 1 cup milk or water
- pinch of salt and cinnamon
- maple syrup, or a different sweetener, to taste
- 1 cup frozen berries of choice or smoothie leftovers

Toppings:

Yogurt

Berries

Directions:

1. In a jar with a lid, add the oats, seeds, milk, salt, and cinnamon, refrigerate overnight. On serving day, puree the berries in a blender.
2. Stir the oats, add in the berry puree and top with yogurt and more berries, nuts, honey, or garnish of your choice. Enjoy!

Nutrition:

Calories:405

Carbs: 65g

Fat: 11g

Protein: 17g

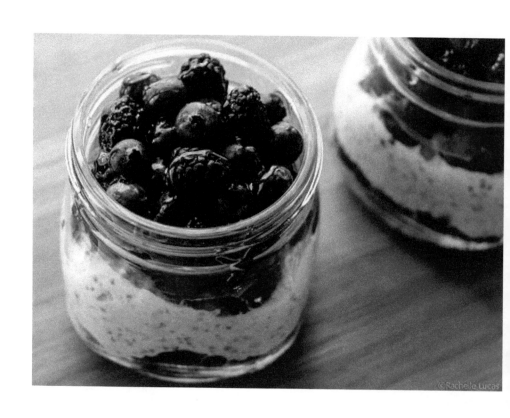

Mango Pear Smoothie

Preparation Time: 5 minutes

Cooking Time: 0 minute

Servings: 1

Ingredients:

- 2 ice cubes
- ½ cup Greek yogurt, plain
- ½ mango, peeled, pitted & chopped
- 1 cup kale, chopped
- 1 pear, ripe, cored & chopped

Directions:

1. Take all ingredients and place them in your blender. Blend together until thick and smooth. Serve.

Nutrition:

Calories 350

Protein 40g

Fats 12g

Carbohydrates: 11 g

Beans, Grains, and Pastas

Chard and Mushroom Risotto

Prep time: 15 minutes | Cook time: 20 minutes | Serves 4

3 tablespoons olive oil

1 onion, chopped

2 Swiss chard, stemmed and chopped

1 cup risotto rice

$\frac{1}{3}$ cup white wine

3 cups vegetable stock

½ teaspoon salt

½ cup mushrooms

4 tablespoons pumpkin seeds, toasted

$\frac{1}{3}$ cup grated Pecorino Romano cheese

1. Heat oil on Sauté, and cook onion and mushrooms for 5 minutes, stirring, until tender. Add the rice and cook for a minute. Stir in wine and cook for 2 to 3 minutes until almost evaporated.
2. Pour in stock and season with salt. Seal the lid and cook on High Pressure for 10 minutes. Do a quick release. Stir in chard until wilted, mix in cheese to melt, and serve scattered with pumpkin seeds.

Per Serving

calories: 420 | fat: 17.7g | protein: 11.8g | carbs: 54.9g | fiber: 4.9g | sodium: 927mg

Cheesy Tomato Linguine

Prep time: 15 minutes | Cook time: 11 minutes | Serves 4

2 tablespoons olive oil

1 small onion, diced

2 garlic cloves, minced

1 cup cherry tomatoes, halved

1½ cups vegetable stock

¼ cup julienned basil leaves

1 teaspoon salt

½ teaspoon ground black pepper

¼ teaspoon red chili flakes

1 pound (454 g) Linguine noodles, halved

Fresh basil leaves for garnish

½ cup Parmigiano-Reggiano cheese, grated

1. Warm oil on Sauté. Add onion and Sauté for 2 minutes until soft. Mix garlic and tomatoes and sauté for 4 minutes. To the pot, add vegetable stock, salt, julienned basil, red chili flakes and pepper.

2. Add linguine to the tomato mixture until covered. Seal the lid and cook on High Pressure for 5 minutes.

3. Naturally release the pressure for 5 minutes. Stir the mixture to ensure it is broken down.

4. Divide into plates. Top with basil and Parmigiano-Reggiano cheese and serve.

Per Serving

calories: 311 | fat: 11.3g | protein: 10.3g | carbs: 42.1g | fiber: 1.9g | sodium: 1210mg

Beef and Bean Stuffed Pasta Shells

Prep time: 15 minutes | Cook time: 17 minutes | Serves 4

2 tablespoons olive oil

1 pound (454 g) ground beef

1 pound (454 g) pasta shells

2 cups water

15 ounces (425 g) tomato sauce

1 (15-ounce / 425-g) can black beans, drained and rinsed

15 ounces (425 g) canned corn, drained (or 2 cups frozen corn)

10 ounces (283 g) red enchilada sauce

4 ounces (113 g) diced green chiles

1 cup shredded Mozzarella cheese

Salt and ground black pepper to taste

Additional cheese for topping

Finely chopped parsley for garnish

1. Heat oil on Sauté. Add ground beef and cook for 7 minutes until it starts to brown.
2. Mix in pasta, tomato sauce, enchilada sauce, black beans, water, corn, and green chiles and stir to coat well. Add more water if desired.

3. Seal the lid and cook on High Pressure for 10 minutes. Do a quick Pressure release. Into the pasta mixture, mix in Mozzarella cheese until melted; add black pepper and salt. Garnish with parsley to serve.

Per Serving

calories: 1006 | fat: 30.0g | protein: 53.3g | carbs: 138.9g | fiber: 24.4g | sodium: 1139mg

Caprese Fusilli

Prep time: 15 minutes | Cook time: 7 minutes | Serves 3

1 tablespoon olive oil

1 onion, thinly chopped

6 garlic cloves, minced

1 teaspoon red pepper flakes

2½ cups dried fusilli

1 (15-ounce / 425-g) can tomato sauce

1 cup tomatoes, halved

1 cup water

¼ cup basil leaves

1 teaspoon salt

1 cup Ricotta cheese, crumbled

2 tablespoons chopped fresh basil

1. Warm oil on Sauté. Add red pepper flakes, garlic and onion and cook for 3 minutes until soft.
2. Mix in fusilli, tomatoes, half of the basil leaves, water, tomato sauce, and salt. Seal the lid, and cook on High Pressure for 4 minutes. Release the pressure quickly.
3. Transfer the pasta to a serving platter and top with the crumbled ricotta and remaining chopped basil.

Per Serving

calories: 589 | fat: 17.7g | protein: 19.5g | carbs: 92.8g | fiber: 13.8g | sodium: 879mg

Chicken and Spaghetti Ragù Bolognese

Prep time: 15 minutes | Cook time: 42 minutes | Serves 8

2 tablespoons olive oil

6 ounces (170 g) bacon, cubed

1 onion, minced

1 carrot, minced

1 celery stalk, minced

2 garlic cloves, crushed

¼ cup tomato paste

¼ teaspoon crushed red pepper flakes

1½ pounds (680 g) ground chicken

½ cup white wine

1 cup milk

1 cup chicken broth

Salt, to taste

1 pound (454 g) spaghetti

1. Warm oil on Sauté. Add bacon and fry for 5 minutes until crispy.
2. Add celery, carrot, garlic and onion and cook for 5 minutes until fragrant. Mix in red pepper flakes and tomato paste, and cook for 2 minutes. Break chicken into small pieces and place in the pot.

3. Cook for 10 minutes, as you stir, until browned. Pour in wine and simmer for 2 minutes. Add chicken broth and milk. Seal the lid and cook for 15 minutes on High Pressure. Release the pressure quickly.

4. Add the spaghetti and stir. Seal the lid, and cook on High Pressure for another 5 minutes.

5. Release the pressure quickly. Check the pasta for doneness. Taste, adjust the seasoning and serve hot.

Per Serving

calories: 477 | fat: 20.6g | protein: 28.1g | carbs: 48.5g | fiber: 5.3g | sodium: 279mg

Parmesan Squash Linguine

Prep time: 15 minutes | Cook time: 5 minutes | Serves 4

1 cup flour

2 teaspoons salt

2 eggs

4 cups water

1 cup seasoned breadcrumbs

½ cup grated Parmesan cheese, plus more for garnish

1 yellow squash, peeled and sliced

1 pound (454 g) linguine

24 ounces (680 g) canned seasoned tomato sauce

2 tablespoons olive oil

1 cup shredded Mozzarella cheese

Minced fresh basil, for garnish

1. Break the linguine in half. Put it in the pot and add water and half of salt. Seal the lid and cook on High Pressure for 5 minutes. Combine the flour and 1 teaspoon of salt in a bowl. In another bowl, whisk the eggs and 2 tablespoons of water. In a third bowl, mix the breadcrumbs and Mozzarella cheese.

2. Coat each squash slices in the flour. Shake off excess flour, dip in the egg wash, and dredge

in the bread crumbs. Set aside. Quickly release the pressure. Remove linguine to a serving bowl and mix in the tomato sauce and sprinkle with fresh basil. Heat oil on Sauté and fry breaded squash until crispy.

3. Serve the squash topped Mozzarella cheese with the linguine on side.

Per Serving

calories: 857 | fat: 17.0g | protein: 33.2g | carbs: 146.7g | fiber: 18.1g | sodium: 1856mg

Red Bean Curry

Prep time: 10 minutes | Cook time: 24 minutes | Serves 4

½ cup raw red beans

1½ tablespoons cooking oil

½ cup chopped onions

1 bay leaf

½ tablespoon grated garlic

¼ tablespoon grated ginger

¾ cup water

1 cup fresh tomato purée

½ green chili, finely chopped

¼ teaspoon turmeric

½ teaspoon coriander powder

1 teaspoon chili powder

1 cup chopped baby spinach

Salt, to taste

Boiled white rice or quinoa, for serve

1. Add the oil and onions to the Instant Pot. Sauté for 5 minutes.
2. Stir in ginger, garlic paste, green chili and bay leaf. Cook for 1 minute, then add all the spices.
3. Add the red beans, tomato purée and water to the pot.

4. Cover and secure the lid. Turn its pressure release handle to the sealing position.
5. Cook on the Manual function with High Pressure for 15 minutes.
6. After the beep, do a Natural release for 20 minutes.
7. Stir in spinach and cook for 3 minutes on the Sauté setting.
8. Serve hot with boiled white rice or quinoa.

Per Serving

calories: 159 | fat: 5.6g | protein: 6.8g | carbs: 22.5g | fiber: 5.5g | sodium: 182mg

CPSIA information can be obtained
at www.ICGtesting.com
Printed in the USA
LVHW081117300621
690925LV00048B/297